DISSOCIATIVE IDENTITY DISORDER A GIFT

DISSOCIATIVE IDENTITY DISORDER
A GIFT

U R IDEAL

First published by Amazon in 2013.

Copyright © U R Ideal 2013

All rights reserved. No part of this publication may be reproduced, stored in a retrieval system or transmitted in any form whether that be electronic, mechanical, photocopying, recording or otherwise without the prior written permission of both the copyright owner and the publisher.

ACKNOWLEDGEMENTS

I dedicate this book to my husband and children with love. Thank you to my daughter for designing the front cover. Many thanks to Simon and John. A special thank you to my legal team. I would like to thank my friends who have been so supportive.

What is Dissociative Identify Disorder?

This is the new name for Multiple Personality Disorder. Dissociative Identity is when different personalities are created as a consequence of severe trauma. Dissociative Identity Disorder is usually caused by neglect, emotional abuse, physical abuse and sexual abuse. In five percent of cases it is caused by medical trauma. An alter is one of the many personalities. The different alters have different functions. Alters switch under stress or particular triggers.

Symptoms of D.I.D.

Amnesia

Completely forgetting and being unaware of things. You might meet someone then have no recollection of having met them. It is very frustrating. I try and keep track of what I'm supposed to be doing by writing on the calendar. Unfortunately it doesn't always work as sometimes an alter appears and goes and does something else. People are often upset with you and you have no idea why.

Depression

In my case I have double depression. It is very common to have suicidal thoughts. In my case this has been a persistent thought for quite some time. Suicide attempts are quite common. Because of the alters one usually alerts someone that you are in danger. With therapy and time things will get better.

Anxiety

Because I also suffer from severe Post-traumatic Stress Disorder which most of

these patients do, I have extreme anxiety at times. At times it is so bad that I have to resort to going on Valium temporarily.
Other times I visit the Doctor and he manages to calm me down.

Insomnia

Many patients have terrible trouble sleeping. In my case sleeping tablets didn't work. In the end I saw a sleep specialist who consulted with my Psychiatrist and they realized I had double depression. My Psychiatrist put me on medication for the double depression that solved the insomnia problem instantly.

Hearing Voices

With this disorder you hear internal voices. The alters all have internal conversations with each other. It can be irritating at times, other times it can be quite comforting. During the day if they all argue with each other I put the radio on to stop them. It distracts them all and gives me a break from it. Sometimes the amount of mental activity going on in my head is too much and I end up with headaches from the stress of it all.

Using Different Names

In my case I have a history of using names that are not my birth name. This has led to some funny and not so funny revelations.

Alcoholism

Alcohol is often used as an escape. Alcohol is used as a coping mechanism. The only problem is it quickly leads to further problems. Addiction and making depression worse and if you are lucky you do rehab.

Coping with D.I.D.

Most of these people also have PTSD and Borderline Personality Disorder. The symptoms of PTSD are flashbacks, nightmares and anxiety. If you know what triggers your PTSD you can try and avoid these situations to try and keep the PTSD under control. Symptoms of Borderline Personality Disorder are impulsive and risky behaviour, self-harm, mood swings,anxiety, depression, inability to control emotions and suicidal behaviour. There is no form of medication for D.I.D. Having said that though some patients do go on medication to treat anxiety, depression or both. Also some patients have co-existing disorders for e.g. Bipolar disorder. The best treatment for Dissociative Identity Disorder is long term Psychotherapy.

Dealing with Dr's, Counsellors, Psychologists and Psychiatrists

You are going to need a very understanding G.P. I went through a number of Doctors until I found the one I currently have. Luckily for me my Doctor specialises in Psychological medicine and believes in the existence of D.I.D. Surprisingly not all Psychiatrists believe in D.I.D. I have seen many Counsellors and Psychologists all who unfortunately managed to seriously destabilise me by retraumatising me.

My Psychiatrist does not ask me to continually go over old traumatic material. This was the mistake all the other clinicians made. My Psychiatrist and Doctor work together in a shared care arrangement. Some Psychologists and Psychiatrists wish to integrate all of the alters into one personality. This really is a decision that needs to be made by the patient.

In my case I am working towards greater communication and agreement between the alters. I am hoping for co-consciousness between all the alters. At present I suffer from blank spells where I don't know what happened.

How D.I.D. Is Portrayed In The Media Compared To Reality?

People with this disorder are often portrayed as serial murderers and disturbed individuals. In rare cases this may be true but most people with this disorder are quite normal.
The alters are still the same person just from different ages and stages of their life. The way I would describe it is the person with Dissociative Identity Disorder goes back in time but no-one else does. My family says it's so interesting living with me they don't need to watch telly.
So called normal people are most often the people with the most disturbing behaviour.

Hypnosis

It is easy to hypnotize someone with D.I.D. I think it would be most unwise to agree to be hypnotized if you have D.I.D. Due to lack of trust these patients need to feel in control of themselves.

Choosing A Therapist

Do choose someone who understands about D.I.D. If the first person you see is no good try someone else. You will have being blocking your feelings by using alters. You will gradually get in touch with your feelings. You will experience all sorts of negative emotions before you start to feel better. You will also need a crisis plan in place.

Dissociating

Apparently I am so good at dissociating that at times specialists have thought I wasn't dissociating when clearly I was.

Hospital Stays

Generally speaking with these patients they should only be hospitalised in really extreme cases. These patients don't like losing control over their lives. In my case because I have suffered medical trauma if I end up in hospital for an overdose they then quickly send me home with my husband. If they admitted me it is likely my condition would further deteriorate due to loss of control.

Is Having D.I.D. A Gift?

Now that I have found out that I have Dissociative Identity Disorder I have decided that it is a Gift. If I didn't have Dissociative Identity Disorder I would most probably be dead. Dissociative Identity Disorder is the brain's way of coping with the unimaginable. Initially I thought I was crazy. The reality is some of my personalities are remarkably normal. Other personalities are not so normal my children just describe me as being "very interesting".

With this disorder people have child, teenage and adult alters. Things can get interesting pretty quickly.

Dissociative Identity Disorder is a complex system that gives the person the ability to function without going crazy. Dissociation is a psychological mechanism to prevent the trauma from being too overwhelming. These individuals have the ability to fit in with anybody and understand anybody due to their ability to see things from many different perspectives. These individuals are geniuses and very creative and often underestimate their own abilities.

At times I have been accused of being psychic. This is probably due to extreme PTSD. All of these patients will tell you that they can always spot a liar a mile away.

People will recognize your problem solving abilities and ask you for advice and support. No matter what problem anyone brings to me I always see it as trivial, not that I tell them that.

A person with Dissociative Identity Disorder is very good at multi-tasking. Usually they will do far more in a day than a normal person except are sometimes unaware of it.

The Gift Of Dissociative Identity Disorder

People with Dissociative Identity Disorder are highly creative and artistic. They tend to paint, write , play musical instruments and are very good at acting. They also achieve things that other people could never even consider. Because your alters all like to do different things people often find you interesting.

Because I have this disorder I have the most outrageous sense of humour. As an aside not you should never play pranks or purposefully upset someone with D.I.D. You should be as kind and considerate as possible. My friends have told me that anyone who has ever upset me has discovered that they messed with the wrong person. Why would you upset someone who has suffered extreme trauma and has more than one hundred personalities. It's like taking on an army of a hundred exceptionally intelligent people. In hindsight it would be the stupidest thing anyone could ever try. Fortunately I never do anything illegal but apparently I do take very clever revenge and never remember having done so. (How embarrassing!)

All of my friends who have this condition also have a very well-developed sense of humour. I actually think it's a built in survival mechanism. Without my sense of humour I just couldn't go on. I even crack jokes and laugh when I'm severely depressed I use it as a coping strategy. I have learned to accept the positive attributes of D.I.D.

Tips For Bad Moments

- Whatever is happening remember it is just temporary and it will pass
- Listen to Music
- Visit a friend
- Go for a walk
- Read
- Write
- Paint
- Watch a comedy
- (Do anything safe that will get you through the next minute, hour, day etc until things improve)
- If you need help, seek help, ring the Samaritans, Dr, Crisis etc
- Keep a Gratitude diary (every day write down at least one thing you are grateful for)

Relaxation

Learn the art of relaxation. Lie down and read a book or listen to relaxing music. Spend some time in the garden. Have a nice soak in a bubble bath. Make sure that you find some relaxation time every day so that things don't get on top of you.

Exercise

If you are suffering from depression or anxiety exercise will help. Daily exercise even if it is just a 30 minute walk every day is very beneficial. I know at one point I was so exhausted I could only make it to the letterbox. I wish I was joking but I am not. Once I got on top of my sleep problem I gradually increased how far I walked. It's amazing how much better you feel after a nice walk. I always feel less anxious and depressed.

Healthy Eating

Try and eat a well-balanced diet. With depression and anxiety you have to be very careful not to fall into the habit of not eating a lot and losing too much weight. Or of no longer caring and constantly eating all the wrong food and gaining too much weight.
You should be eating protein, fruit and vegetables, nuts and a small amount of good quality carbohydrates.

Take Control Of Your Life

Plan in advance. Try not to take on too much. You need to make sure you have plenty of time in your life for rest, relaxation and fun.

Goal Setting

If you are not in a good space right now start off with small goals. Clean out the hall cupboard. Have a friend over for lunch.
As you start to improve set bigger goals. Do you want to change careers? Or do you want to go somewhere different for the holidays?

Expectations

In all honesty there are times when you are just going to need to lower your expectations. If you are feeling awful one night of takeaways or delaying housework is not going to mean the whole world will fall apart. Having said this though you may feel better if one room say the lounge is tidy.

Caring for others
Sometimes if you volunteer and do something for someone else you will feel better about yourself. Do make sure that you look after yourself though. Even if you just pick flowers out of your own garden and put them in a vase in the dining room it may cheer you up. Always remember to pamper yourself it doesn't have to be expensive and you are worth it.

Self-esteem

Always dress well and don't lose interest in hygiene and appearance. Also be very careful of self-talk. Anything you say to yourself should be kind. As Dissociative Identity Disorder patients have persecutor alters you just have to very firmly tell that alter that they are wrong and they need to talk to you nicely. If we don't accept people in our lives being horrible to us we shouldn't let our alters do it either. I know this is easier said than done. This is where playing music comes in handy. You could even get real funny with this and choose a particular song like "You don't always get what you want!"

Friends

You don't have to have thousands of friends or even hundreds. I am very blessed to have some long-term friends I have had since school. I have also made other lovely friends along the way. It is more important to me that I have genuine friends. I would far rather have less friends and for them to be real than to have lots of those fake friends people seem to have nowadays.

All of my friends have stood by me through thick and thin. It can't have been easy at times either. One of my friends said, "I don't know how such an intelligent woman can get into so much trouble in such a short space of time?" This particular friend had begun to suspect I had D.I.D. A month later I worked it out.

My friends have been very supportive of my condition. They all say I am the same person that I always was. It hasn't changed how any of them feel towards me. They all still love and care about me. They said it just explains a few things they couldn't quite understand before.

I am quite open about my diagnosis. In my case my Dissociative Identity Disorder has been caused by Medical Trauma. I don't have to worry about it harming my career prospects as I work as an author. My children are teenagers and they know about the diagnosis as do some of their friends. My children and their friends just find me very interesting. I think the more people talk about conditions like this the more people will understand it and it will demystify people's beliefs about D.I.D.

Printed in Great Britain
by Amazon